NB: *The author thanks in advance the readers for their indulgence with regard to certain short-comings of the translation. Knowing that this will not interfere with the importance of the book's content. Your comments will be welcomed. Contact the author on the Internet at* **''Amazon''- "My Evil is a Calvary"** *- leaving a comment and a mail address.*

MY EVIL
IS
A CALVARY

Translated from French
By René D. LA PLANETA

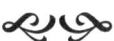

Hell of Verneuil's disease
(Hidradenitis Suppurativa)

By

Doriane GOHAUD
and
Rene D. LA PLANETA

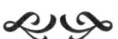

Dedication:

To my family, Mom, my sister Anne-Sophie, my nephew Maxence and my niece Solène, so full of attentions, Farid my companion; To all my friends for their self-sacrifice for the comfort of their unwavering support since the beginning of my hell.

A mention for Celine Kuzik, my friend in difficult times, which was me great moral support despite her own difficulties.

To all those whom a blind destiny has struck with this calamity represented by the Verneuil's disease. May they find, by my words, the reflection of the suffering they endure, and that they cannot communicate because of lack of audience. My wish is to give them, by my personal testimony, a complement of courage that they already show in the face of the ordeal with which they suffer in silence, and often in isolation, for it is true that our humanity tends to stand far away of those who suffer and weep as if afraid of contagion.

May my brothers and sisters victims of the same sufferings, share with me the hope that soon our existence of damned will end.

Doriane GOHAUD

Author:

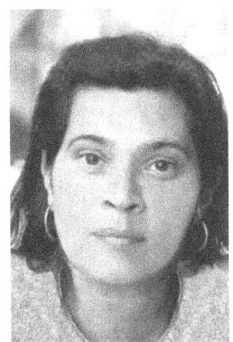 Doriane Gohaud was born in region of Paris on October 13, 1965. After a traditional elementary education, having few attractions for the school, she wanted quickly to start a professional activity. Having always been interested in the desire to be useful and to serve, her choice has been directed towards the assistance of the destitute, and the defenseless poor people of our humanity. To this end, she trained herself in accommodation and supervision facilities for people with intellectual disabilities, before turning to the disabled and poly-disabled. The discovery of this population and the distress it endures, has decided of her vocation. Using the support of her mother, secretary at ADAPEI[1] Valfleury, in the county of Loire *(France)*, she could, at the age of eighteen, take the service of the forgotten of our humanity. In spite of the difficulties of the function, despite the constraints of a difficult and sometimes repulsive work, she flourishes in the sense of happiness that bring the devotion to our

---

[1] *ADAPEI: Organization for the assistance to intellectually defective persons.*

fellowmen. It was with the courage and obstinacy of an ant that she pursued her mission, when destiny manifested itself by striking her with the terrible and incurable abomination of Verneuil's disease. This did not prevent her from continuing her work despite the pain and disability. It is the result of her own ordeal and the discovery of the abandonment of the victims of this terrible scourge, who decided her to testify by writing this book with the help of a friend of her family. His book reveals the existence of a world of sufferings and horrors that we encounter every day without our being aware of it; It is a call to those whose heart cannot remain indifferent to the fate of millions of children, women and men *(estimated at more than 4% of the world's population)* who have seen their lives destroyed by the insidious plague that represents the Verneuil's disease...

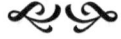

*... I have come to sing my pain and shout
to passers-by to call the sympathy of
the most distant unknowns ...*

Pierre LOTI - French Author
(The novel of a child)

Prologue:

Most of us believe that life is a common thing that everyone gets fairly. I shared this point of view for a long time, which seemed logical. A quiet youth, under a sky that has not known heavy clouds, comforted me in this belief that existence, indulgent and just, gave everyone an equal opportunity. Nothing around me suggesting the opposite, I have made myself to this type of philosophy. The story I am going to confide to these pages, will contradict, unfortunately, this preconceived idea, demonstrating, if necessary, that nothing is more capricious and incoherent than the creation, for which equity is the last preoccupation. Without rebel against a state of things against which I can't do anything, I wonder, sometimes, however, why, this lottery of the fate that intervene and blindly hit humans, treated like game objects. It sometimes happens a question that often arises to those born under the aegis of a bad star, *"Why me? ..."*

CHAPTER I

Once upon a time...

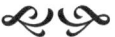

Once upon a time ... It is with these words that always start stories. In the manner of a ship majestically leaving port to begin a long journey, life takes off in the cradle, the difference between the humans being that it reveals only our trip starting point; masking its final destination and, even more, the state of the ocean on which it will make us sail. It has its moods; sometimes mild, sometimes furious. Our lives, as well, are in dependence of its whims. This one will make an idyllic cruising where another will encounter demented storms. Heralding the beginnings of storms is frequently absent, leaving us at the mercy of the elements, without the possibility of guard against the evils of the coming tempest. Thus I entered into existence by a sunny day when all seemed serene. - On October 13, 1965, at the fall line, in the Paris region, arrived on earth a charming little girl who received from her parents' the first name of Doriane that his buddies teens turn into "DOD". Little face at the bottom of a cradle, that baby was me. Nothing really distinguished me from other children born the same day, having opened their eyes to the world in ignorance of what would be their fate...

I was, it seems, adorable, although this view can be relativized, because it was issued by my parents whose opinion, like for all parents, might be tainted by bias, as is known. My first two years of existence passed without problems, surrounded by the affection of my family. Alas, as I reached my two and a half years, for reasons of its own, Dad left us, Mom and me, which forced us to go stay with my maternal grandparents who lived in northern France, in quite a different environment. I do not really felt the immediate effects of subsequent changes to the separation of the authors of my days, probably because of my age. Yet I remember, as surprising as it may seem, of this first upheaval in my life. Although negative, this change brought a compensation came from the overflowing affection of my grandparents, for whom, from the day I was born, I had become the navel of the world. Despite all the attention which I was the center, I did, I am told, a small depression. I knew, a little later, the experience of early education in a religious institution, whose the only notable reminiscences relate to the abundance of tears I kept pouring.

Mom was still at this time in the spring of life; she met a gentleman, a little younger than she, who in the logic of things, at some point became my second dad. Youth of the newlyweds eventually bear fruit, and so is in the middle of the summer of 1971, on July 2, that the reconstituted family welcomed a little sister who was called Anne-Sophie. I was happy to get out of my solitude with the arrival of the new baby that I was delighted to welcome. Our age difference soon led me to consider the baby as a new doll, offering the privilege of saying early *"Daddy"*, *"Mom,"* and, wonder of wonders, to pee herself in bed without it being necessary to fill it with water such as trade baby toys .

My second dad treated me in my early youth as his own daughter. Due to professional constraints, we had to leave the north of France to settle in Sorbiers, a nice little village in the county of Loire near the city of Saint-Etienne, in the south of the country. This move was penalized by the loss of all relations with neighbors who, in the land of *"Ch'tis²"*, was the equivalent of a second family. As for me, the event saddened me because of the break with my grandparents that I cherished, and whose tenderness was beyond

---

² *Name given in France to the inhabitants of the North.*

the possible. But as nothing is irreversible, although limited, arrangements were made for that only two or three times a year, I may know the joy of reunion with this Grandpa and Grandma that I loved deeply. In this beautiful region of Saint-Etienne with significant natural resources, we organized us to multiply the excursions along the Loire River, such as *"barbecue days"*, where we could fun playing the new Robinsons.

Life is not embarrassed with considerations, I adapt to my new existence with joyful recklessness that characterizes children of my age of this time. Full of health and energy, I enrolled in the club *"L'Arc-en-Ciel[3]"* there to practice gymnastics, sports that I was involved with an energy that allowed me to shine there. My little sister followed in the wake, which allowed me to play a little at a den mother, without, however, it put a shadow over our good friendship. This chieftain temperament was, I think, be a part of my profile if I judge from the opinion of my friends at the time who, despite everything, endured me with amiable patience perhaps because I always was arranging to choose them younger than me. Thus I can say that my childhood was not unhappy without, however, say

---

[3] *"The rainbow"*

that it was happy. However, something was simmering, which took shape when I entered the time of adolescence. After the death of my maternal grandparents, who made me very sorry because they have always been for me a part of my sunshine, the attitude of my stepfather changed from a quiet tolerance to an authoritarianism going crescendo. The thing at a time, turned to a real persecution where, by the authority conferred to him by his right of family head, he began to harass me, passing his moods on me, forbidding me attendance of my friends, opposing the least of my outings, putting his veto to all my escape attempts in activities likely to withdraw me from his authority.

Although I could not complain of displaced gestures, this new state had intervened in my life making me a true recluse, until I reach my majority, where I resumed the disposal of my person, with the blessing of my mother, who did not intervened, not by   fear, but to preserve the semblance of harmony that reigned at home, making of her the impotent witness of my stress.

With a cheerful nature, I have always expressed an interest in the people around me. As already said, I don't like school, and especially college; which led me to quickly search an escape in the work, which led me to enroll in a women's hairdressing apprenticeship course. I passed successfully, though without conviction, my PAC[4] hairdresser and I walked into a salon. The days at the hair salon soon became a burdensome activity, during which I had to listen with feigned sympathy that was painful to me, about the superficial and boring small talk of Mrs Down, clients of the shop, who saw me as a privileged audience at their disposal. My majority bringing me the free disposal of myself, I started looking for a job in line with my expectations. Having heard of people with disabilities, I prospected in that direction. My first contact with this medium enlightened me on what would be my vocation: "educator with disabled people." Be helpful to others, there had to establish my future.

My parents had a house built in the Valfleury region, still in the county of Loire; I had to face a new break with my environment. New comer in the new environment, no more friends, no more sports club, in short a new state of isolation. But the thing did not last; with a communicative nature I soon managed to restore my relations from which was formed a small gang which became the remedy to my crisis of melancholy. Employing Sioux tricks, thanks to the complicity

---

[4] *PAC : Certificate of Apprenticeship.*

of the others, I managed to attend my first ball. It was time to explore the sentimental emotions. In the manner of children tales of princesses, I had the impression of entering an unknown realm, with its happiness, its dreams and other marvels. As often noted, additional difficulties overcome, gave spice to the thing, placing my experiences of this period at the forefront of the beautiful memories of my youth.

An event of great importance for me was, however, marked this period of my life: My Stepfather, although barely forty-two, died of cancer consecutive to the abuse of alcohol and tobacco. With the risk that I could be considered an insensitive, I felt this death as a liberation, although it was sad for my little sister, who was touched by the death of her real dad. Near our new home, was a host institution for people with intellectual disabilities. Luck and chance meant that my mother, professional secretary, found a position in the institution that recognized her merits, allowing her to quickly take responsibilities.

With the help of references acquired in some institutions for intellectual handicapped in 1984, ADAPEI recruiting staff, I was engaged in a position that would quickly become a profession; My job.

All events occurred had transformed our lives. We now had a home where love prevailed among the three women who occupied it: My mother, my sister, and myself. Another happy going to happen, I met the man who would become my companion. The poor did not know at that time what was going to cost him, of dedication and self-sacrifice, his love for me. But I will come back on this point later.

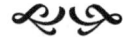

CHAPTER II

A world of Aliens

Although I arrived at ADAPEI at a very young age and trained in institutions for the disabled, it was for me a discovery and a deep emotion. I was overwhelmed with confused feelings. The loss marks in my relationships with my new patients and deep sorrow at the situation they were in. The term conditions, needless to say, does not refer here to a material situation or comfort because, in this regard, the establishment and its specialized staff offered what was best. ; I talk about my feelings in front of people belonging to a world so different from the one I knew. My emotion was profound when I was in contact with young beings *(Some were my age)* than their mental difficulties locked up in a world apart. I keep the memory of a young autistic angelic face, which upset me by putting on me a look full of sweetness and intelligence, which I could not answer, in the absence of a language adapted to our communication.

Like many of our fellow men, my ignorance made me imagine the world of intellectual inadequacies such as people living in a vegetative state deprived of all humanity. What was my astonishment to discover living beings, with attention and sometimes endearing outbursts like children's gestures. Vulnerable beings and devoid of malice to which I attached myself spontaneously. As you may have noticed, I have not used the term handicapped or mentally retarded; it does not fit them. As confirm all those who work in contact with them, they are eminently social and keen to do well. Even those that affect extreme deficiencies, life is there, present; I would be tempted to say, "*Lurking*", as if they were trying to escape from their tower of silence at the slightest flash of lucidity.

I discovered later the world of those who, at the extreme point of disability, were in a state of complete absence and had to be completely take over. In the moment I admired the courage and dedication of the exceptional degree of personnel responsible for the painful task of their accompaniment. Young devoted women whose ungrateful work they accept remain ignored by most of us. Although they would show in astonished if told them; they are the guardian angels of those men, women and children, affected by the vagaries of blind and indifferent nature, if not ruthless.

I finished my training of instructor educator in 1992, and failed, unfortunately, to my graduation. The financial requirements of life put me under obligation to enter without waiting in the world of work. Despite my failure to graduation of instructor, the training received and experience with people with disabilities who sought me with a skill, I obtained a CSD at the village of Saint-Exupéry Red-Cross, City of Saint-Chamond, Loire. My experience allowed me a rapid integration within healthcare teams of the organization. The colleagues I met there were a great help to me in my adaptation. I owe them for teaching me what could be called the ABC of trade. With unfailing patience, they introduced to me the care of people with multiple disabilities in all acts of daily life: Get up, eat, walk, wash, with the inescapable and binding set of corporal needs. This assistance was all the more precious to me than my actual achievements were at the level of the experience associated with my stay at the Intellectually Handicapped, during my training as an instructor educator. The people I was talking about at the time belonged to a group that spent an essential part of its time at CAT[5].

---

[5] *CAT : Help Center by Work*

The people I told about at that time belonged to a group spending an essential part of his time in CAT[6].

The center designed to train people with disabilities, providing them with professional knowledge suitable to leading them, in the best case, to an autonomy. I filled them with an educational role in accompanying their daily lives. Some of my patients were affected by multiple disabilities denying them any autonomy. Many were undergoing wheelchairs, enduring moreover, the constraints of a rigid corset. The extent of these types of disabilities makes it particularly difficult assistance work associated with these people. The organization gathered in the *"Groups of life"* with six patients that attend nursing aids and AMP[7], expected to take full care of the residents.

The novelty of the work distraught at first, as born from the difficulty to communicate with the people entrusted to our care. We feel destabilized and even helpless by their inability to express themselves verbally, but also physically, by gestures, just by issuing these elementary signals that represent a smile or a simple mimicry; making all things complex detection of their needs

---

[6] *CAT : Help Center by Work*
[7] *AMP: Medical and Psychological Assistant*

and expectations, because of our inability to read a message on sometimes faces deprived of any expression. In the long run, this destabilizes caregivers who gnaw their gray matter in questions about *"Does he (Or she) understand what I try to tell him?" Does it hurt somewhere? Is she suffers? "Has she or, has he need something?"* These are grueling situations, if not exhausting in the long run. The Assistants are required to deploy ingenuity to break the silence and to enter into the closed world of their patients, some of whom were not even aware of the world around them. Especially because each case is specific. One could say that disabilities are followed and are not alike; each providing its survival on its own resources. Beyond stress and psychological tension, personal care and assistance centers for people with disabilities is seen, moreover, confronted with the physical effort imposed by frequent handling that they need to operate on their patients.

The difficulties of our profession are however mitigated by the solidarity and the spirit of cooperation that prevails among colleagues working on what are called *"living groups".* This term refers to people whose daily lives are not suspected by the outside world. Ignoring what can be experienced by those who are responsible for their well-being in a world far from the common. It is these peculiarities that make our work exciting despite his fatigue and exhausting side.

The exciting term is justified by the constant questioning of professional practice, following the changing behavior of unstable patients in permanent evolution. If the management of Mr, or Ms. "X" went well one day, there is no guarantee that it will be the same the next day. The subjects in our care have their own profiles that require taken them into specific care. Particularities linked to routes to the origin of their arrival in the center; whether their lives, their environment or of their medical course. The people concerned are often "*placed*" because of their particular situation; for their good, you can hear it. Many are very young at their entry into *(M.E.I Medical-Educational Institute)* and in the dependence of an evolving handicap. There I happened to see residents join the *Saint-Exupéry-Village* Centre enjoying their independence movements with the use of a walker, finding them, a few years later, in a wheelchair. Thus our workload gets heavier by complications, due to the lack of additional staff, assigned to specialized tasks allowing the continuity of the quality of care.

The situation of the patients varies with social origin. It is not a question necessarily of the concept of income but of educational level or cultural background. Thus I am currently working with six residents with a similar state of consciousness, but accusing substantial differences in age of about twenty years. Clearly, their tastes vary accordingly and, this one, for fun, appreciate listening to a singer as *"taylor SWIFT"* or *"Dylan O'BRIEN"*, will not share the pleasure of those who lean to *"Frank SINATRA"* or *"Barbara STREISAND"*. It's the same for all activities, from trips to the choice of clothes or food. Our mission is to help satisfying from our best; these differences in expectations is sometimes for us a real Chinese puzzle, especially as our use of resources are inevitably limited.

Other differences, some people are able to use wheelchairs propelled by the use of one or both hands *(They are called "Manual")*, capable of a certain autonomy in terms of one or both arms. This ability can be exploited by the play of reflexes, and can often be completed by piloting motorized wheelchairs with electric motors. Thereof, requiring intellectual resources imposing the ability to discriminate between press a "button" to start, and prolonging the action by the use of a "joystick" to manage the path and movement speed of the chair. The intellectual failure of pilot would quickly transform the corridors of the center in bumper cars track.

Besides the *"autonomous"*, quadriplegics are completely unable to move, in any form whatsoever. This does not exclude, for some, the ability to hear, see, and understand, in a perfect state of consciousness. These unfortunates, absolutely unable to move, would be condemned to a purely vegetative existence in the absence of a support by an alternate person to ambulatory their shortcomings; otherwise, they would remain there in the passivity of a simple object, such as vegetables at the bottom of a pantry. With our support, those who see and hear retain the privilege of escaping a few moments watching TV, or the spectacle of the outer life by being placed in front of a window. Among their popular recreations include meals and time to the toilet which, for a few brief moments, give them sensations that bring them the feeling of existing.

In the moments when my morale takes a break, I am delighted to have chosen the job I'm doing, thinking that if I had chosen a job filling of yoghurt pots in *"Mountain High"*, I would had not the heart to go to work the days I am crossing deserts of my pain. Maybe I would have increased my sick leave. Perhaps would I have had fewer scruples about feeling sorry for myself my feelings, leaving my colleagues lonely face to their machines. Today, I am sure that I owe to my professional occupations to have forged the character with which I overcome my ordeal. More than once, I happened to tell me: *"My little Dod, you complain, when these poor people do not even have time to be able to speak of their suffering or even scratch their noses when they itches them... So stop complaining and whining!"*- I comfort me in parallel with the fact that if I'm not always able to dress myself, I retain the privilege of walking or tapping away on a computer keyboard. Sometimes, I cannot drive or go out for my liking, but I can call friends on the phone when my loneliness becomes too unbearable. I realize that these are the privileges that help me fight. The practice of a tough job, sometimes challenging, is to me an advantage, and I do not regret having chosen it. When I go to my work, I don't anticipate the difficulties that await me with *"the knot in my stomach."* I know that difficult times will be at the Rendezvous, but it stimulates me instead of discouraging me. I do not despair, when I will cross the threshold of a late career, to see me entrust more autonomous individuals, allowing reports of greater intellectual intensity and less physically exhausting.

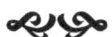

CHAPTER III

The land of the forgotten

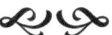

I open my eyes after a restless night; a dull day filters through the shutters; the atmosphere is gloomy. I get up and open the window; early winter mottled with snow the landscape; Ice crystals glittering on branches of the trees, spread in a thin white coat herald the coming of Christmas. This postcard setting back a little morale and it is with some enthusiasm that I conduct my toilet. After a comfortable breakfast demanded by the day that awaits me, I put on my coat and gloves, before going to take possession of my car waiting for me outside my door quietly, huddled under its blanket of snow. This coat will be my first act of the year by the inauguration of the daily routine, with ten to fifteen minutes imposed scraping frost covering my windows and my windshield.

On the road, the flock coating is still superficial; to paraphrase the poet, winter has covered the decor with white powdered hair, wrapping the landscape with a white frosty veil. The post-card is ready and were it not unlike the color of my clothes, I could take me for a pixie of my child-hood fables that have grown too much. I drive with caution because if the snow is not thick, it is completely frozen and it would take little for my car is tempted by the drunken skater step of a double axel. I am fortunate to live in the country-side, surrounded by trees and greenery. In little more than a hundred meters from my home, I walked along a pasture where a herd of horses frolics; this is one of my favorite moments. The animals are adorable; their dresses are in shiny wiry hair in this season. Their colors are beauti-ful, the dark bay dapple gray, passing through the jet black, white and cherry. They interest me so much that I went to inform me about them. I watch them frolic, indifferent to temperature, they roll on the ground by emitting small neigh-ing of fun that would make think of laughs. I love them because they are for me the image of what I love more: *"Freedom"*. If I were like them, they would be in the fields, while I would stay con-fined in a box by an evil that obscures me. - Still rolling, I cross the city of Saint-Chamond still bit choppy at this time. Having recovered from my bad night I drive mechanically, like a sleep-walker. I exceed the suburbs to find me, without transition, in the foothills of the *Massif du Pilat*[8]. The road to the *Valla-en-Giers*[9] sinuing among the orchards. The trees, so beautiful in spring, when its awakening covers the fields of flowers, are only at this moment the sad phantoms stripped of their leaves by the arrival of winter. The cherry trees, a specialty of the region, replaced their white petals with a gel implemented by the magic wand of nature. Finally, after twelve kilometers of rural escape, shortly before arriving at the dam of Valla, I left the road to enter, on my right, in the huge car park of my place of work along the two buildings of the institution Saint-Exupéry of the Red Cross, nearly two hundred and fifty meters long.

On the left the children home, while his vis-à-vis hosts adults. I park as usual and then I head to the lobby, where I enter through the sliding glass door that closes the entrance. I cross the great hall on the ground floor with access to service areas, loading me in passing with the bread baskets of breakfast that the baker deposited there each morning. I let my left post lifts reserved for the sick, before taking the grand staircase leading upstairs

---

[8] *Mountainous massif dominating the town of Saint-Etienne*
[9] *Small village near the city of Saint-Chamond*

After my ascent, I head to *"the street"*, as we call a huge corridor reminiscent of the bar connecting the balls forming a dumbbell which divides the *"life groups"*, each hosting twenty-four people. I engage on the left of the corridor, at the end of which are the ones I tend to call *"my parishioners"*, as it is true that I feel towards them as a kind of Pastor. I clothe my tee-shirt with the colors of service before passing into the office part of watchmen and night watchers. We exchange a few words. I see that the fatigue resulting from a long vigil combined with the effects of bad weather has reached the limits of their strong constitution; they are exhausted. It is mechanically that girls perform the usual greetings, as they wait to go to rest. Our team consists of five people, divided into three full-time positions and two part-time positions. We respond daily to the needs of six residents with multiple disabilities, consisting of a group of three men and three women. Our work program takes place from 7:00 to 21:30. At that time, night watchmen, night watchers, careers and AMP, take over, which will last until the arrival of the day shift. The organization plans rotations from 7 am to 2:30 pm, with a possibility from 8 am to 4 pm *(quarter-morning)* or from 2 pm to 9 pm. *(Evening shift)*. Our schedules do not include meal times *(What we must to accept).* Our workload makes us often need to refrain from eating, especially at night, due to the asymmetric arrangement of the team, consisting of two male operators or female operators in the morning *(except week-End)* and one in the evening. Sometimes we are more numerous, but in this case we are dealing with exceptional situations called *"assisted contracts".* In the morning, I arrive at the workplace, as is the case today, and I take control of the night watchmen.

From the report they make to me of nightly events, at this time I draw an assistance plan that meets the needs of residents. Thus I will consider the incidents after sunset, as the fact that a resident has been ill or has not slept. In that case, I'll see to realize his condition and according to the results found, I will decide, perhaps, the postponement of the time to get dress and to have her breakfast, to grant him or her an additional time, leaving them some complement of rest and sleep. All of these are documented and communicated to the nurse service, to enable her to intervene if necessary. Among forty-eight, our residents are divided into eight groups. In order to give them a sense of independence and freedom, each group has a common room, called *"life center",* with a kitchen, a TV corner with desk, cupboards, and a patio for the summer, to take the meal outdoors.

All of these are documented and communicated to the nurse service, to enable her to intervene if necessary. Among forty-eight, our residents are divided into eight groups. In order to give them a sense of independence and freedom, each group has a common room, called *"life center"*, with a kitchen, a TV corner with desk, cupboards, and a patio for the summer, to take the meal outdoors. The living room is a central element around which fall six individual rooms, each with a fully equipped bathroom. Generally, when I am on duty, residents are still sleeping at the time of my enter in service; except, as is the case now, a resident who needs to go to the toilet and must attend immediately. - Hello Basil ! So I said jokingly to my patient who wriggles on his bed under the pressure of an urgent pee: An emergency? He replied with a nod, taking his hands clasped between his legs. He cannot move but, although deprived of the ability to walk, he retained the ability to standing. Unable to bear it, I'll get the *"lifter[10]"*; after which I harnessed *"the net"* before installing him on a breakthrough-chair that will be used to move him to the toilet bowl where the net will be removed in time of his natural needs. I leave a few moments, to respect his pri-

---

[10] *System for lifting people with a hoist.*

36

vacy and give him time to satisfy his needs, before returning him to his bed by repeating, in reverse, the previous operations. These operations are complicated with people totally disabled completely amorphous, and cannot even sit still. Total when it includes a built-in seat. Handling proves more delicate because, tailor-made corsets envelop them like a real shell. It is important in these particular situations, to ensure that the garment which takes their bodies do not fold, because the slightest outgrowth would result in localized pressure leading, in the short term, skin alteration causing bedsores. Clearly, these unfortunate already have enough difficulties do not overdo it by negligence. One imagines the work of nursing staff when the rigor of hygiene require making their toilet. After a rough cleaning in their bed, the subjects are *(I have no other word)*, manipulated and installed on their chairs after being harnessed in the "net".

Once the lever is put in place, the lifting cables are secured, then hoisting is carried out for transfer to the bathroom where the ablutions take place. Things get complicated with those that cannot be lifted and which have to be led to the pool in the special bed, a kind of tub on wheels that often get stuck in the too narrow spaces leading to the bathrooms...

It's no wonder that the operative are often exhausted after a day of seven hours and half theoretical, but at least eight hours in fact. Paradoxically, I will not fail to surprise by saying that these victims of fate are encouraging me to live.

Despite the atrocious evil I endure, my troubles seem small and unrelated to theirs. It happens to me, watching, trying to imagine what their thoughts are, (for those who have preserved the faculty of consciousness), by being in the state where they are. Especially since the nature of their evil admits of no hope for improvement if not the expectation of a deeper decline. But, back to my arrival at the center; my first task accomplished, I am aware of the "notes" written by my colleagues on the eve of a record book, or calendar, as it is called. This book traces the course of the day. This procedure allows precise monitoring of the behavior of residents and support depending on their state of mind, or the requirement of medical application instructions for specific care, such as the obligation to remain fasting for blood test or at a specified time for a medical appointment. This is a diary for their regular meetings with the Occupational Therapist, Physical Therapist, the various recreational workshops, outings, vacations, and any programs that shape their lives. We also use it to 'calibrate' our own meeting dates, etc... Then comes the preparation of the breakfast which is established according to the tastes of each one. Some ask to bring it to bed, while others prefer the friendly atmosphere of the group. To all those who might ask for the reasons for all these attentions, it should be noted that all these residents are under medical treatment for certain profound intellectual deficiencies, for whom a simple contradiction could trigger a severe agitation or a melancholic prostration, commonly known under the name of depression. It should be noted that the institution strives to maintain a social life for its residents, emphasizing its purpose, which, through material conditions and the environment, is to lead them to a certain autonomy. This policy, deliberate and effective, leads caregivers to keep closer to their Male or Female patients, ensuring a continuation of a close relationship with the families, which remain a sine qua non element of the success of the program. The polyhandicap is a heavy handicap, often at the basis of multiple disorders: breathing - swallowing - withdrawal and muscle. Each form of disorder involving distinct and complementary exercises such as *"Verticalization"*, *"breathing-exercises"*, *"massages"*, whose purpose is jointly curative but also preventive. I finish my time of Service tense and stressed by physical effort, and by my relationships with residents of the establishment which, by repeated contacts, few are pretty integrated into my life, and whose misfortune does not leave me indifferent, although professional manuals strongly advise to avoid such attachment, for reasons easy to understand. Looking at them, thinking of their marginalization in terms of society, I sometimes think, for them and for me, to an old aphorism whose origin is lost: *"When you'll be in distress, ô my friend hide it well, because here man is only interested on those who need nothing ..."*

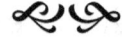

CHAPTER IV

The crossroads of destiny

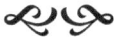

My life took place in serenity conferred by purposeful occupations and feeling of the task performed. The routine basically; all left to think that things would continue as well and that, like all women, one day soon, I would know the joys of motherhood and happiness cries of children accompanying their wild games. We were in 1992 when, without warning, one morning I felt a pain in the groin. This pain is alive, I worried so much more than I was home alone, my companion then being in the south of France for a replacement contract. I felt helpless to deal with my loneliness, I felt shooting pains. However, I grinned and bore it, believing that, from the fact of its sudden appearance, my pain could be only temporary. Contrary to this belief of an uncertain logic, in the day the pain got worse and, concerned about, my mind refuse to spend the next night in its company and in solitude, I did what we all do when we have yet this privilege, I asked Mom to come and share the evening with me. In ignorance of the causes of the evil that I felt, because of its intensity, my second thought was that she could take me to the emergency room if circumstances required.

The next morning I awoke without further alarm, and everything seemed to be back to normal. I was to learn later that the painful thrust was caused by the appearance of a first abscess finally aborted. In the moment, like Cyrano de Bergerac would have said, *"What by the fife comes, goes by the drum"*; causes once disappeared, the effect did the same, my life resumed its course. Several months passed and I was to forget the incident when the disease resumed its offensive. I deliberately use the term *"offensive"* because Verneuil's disease is equivalent to a real war, with its battles, its truces, and the return of its devastating assaults. I will come back to the purely medical aspects of this scourge, but could essentially be called a leprosy and, even better, a real plague whose abscesses are buboes. Often, things begin with a hair follicle who is stuck in his journey toward the skin surface and, accumulating sebum, eventually infect the cells that surround it, creating an abscess; however, this is only one form of the manifestations of the disease. This is where the wanderings of my medical journey will begin. In 1996 my family doctor, alarmed by the recurrence of my abscesses, whose manifestations became more frequent, and in front of my growing anxiety, he sent me to a specialist in Saint Etienne, a professor of dermatology with an established reputation.

Evil evolving, following the painful surges I experienced for the first time, I was compelled twice to a sick leave of several days. I was genuinely sorry because of the attachment I felt for my work on the one hand, for the patients I was in charge of, but also for the impact that this could have on my contract of employment that my absences could compromise. I worked at that time under CDD[11] *(since June 93)* in the town of Saint-Chamond, in the Center Saint-Exupéry, **foster care hospital for adults with multiple disabilities.**

Another concern was mobilizing me: The evolution of my progressive dependence to increasingly strong analgesics, such as *Doliprane* or *Tylenol*, the only remedy that can help me endure my pain, unbearable without them. But as it often happens, as a result of addiction, *Tylenol* soon no longer suffices me, and it gave way to a process of escalation. In the space of four years, I came up with harder drug derivatives based on morphine, such as *Topalgic*.

---

[11] *CDD : Fixed-term contract*

The dermatologist professor whom I had consulted having diagnosed the presence of Staphylococcus aureus, attributed indefinitely to this discovery the responsibility of my boils. So, I found myself in a range of treatments making extensive use of antibiotics which, despite their diversity, the side effects I experienced and the cost, did not change my condition. I began to feel more and more miserable as a result of all these treatments that have become the cause of my suffering. The pleasure I took in contemplating my image in a mirror, like any pretty young woman, is gradually transformed into a nightmare by the discovery of an unknown and wilted skin, ugly as a whole and, for my despair, disgusting. How did it happen? How did it happen? What sin have I committed to deserve such punishment?

Little by little I felt abandoned by a world from which I was gradually excluded by the evil which had seized my body to make it an object of disgust and repulsion. I was fortunate at this stage not to have been struck in the face, the clothes had allowed me to hide my horrors against the wounding glance of the ignorant; but for me, who knew what they were hiding... Through artifices, the patient can mask the effects of the illness, appearing to his entourage like a lazy person when the unbearable pain forces him to suspend work. In 1998 and 1999, I had to increase work stoppages. It was another chance for me, to have, as head of department, an intelligent woman, full of great humanity, capable of understanding what I was enduring. This difficulty for the patients in concealing their state in terms of environment often make them look *"Well and normal"* in appearance, whereas an evil inflicts them its devastation and torture.

Time passes and the specialists consulted continue to be enclosed in a routine type diagnosis *"by Staphylococcus aureus furunculosis"*. In 2000, my general practitioner who does not disarm, sent me to the consultation of another eminent professor of *"infectious department"* of the Bellevue hospital of Saint-Etienne. He was interested in my case and a laudable effort has been made to find a solution. The service goes as far as attempting the realization of a vaccine developed from samples taken from my abscesses. Subsequently, alas, they remained in the traditional; I became again the guinea pig on which one tested different types of antibiotics, with, as the only observable result, side effects depriving me of the small tonus that had not yet left me.

At this moment, the lack of success of the treatments attempted leaves me helpless, faced with the real torture that makes me endure these successive abscesses, appearing in the most unexpected places and, preferably, the most painful of my body: the Armpits, genital and rectal area, breasts, so sensitive in women. Whether we try to imagine what the patient can experience the emergence, in the cited areas, these huge abscess, genuine buboes up to the size of a fist; leaving, like icebergs, flush out the flesh as the fifth or even a tenth of their volume; the eruptions which emptied their boils on the surface of the body converted into a discharge ground for abject purulent sanies, when they do not stink. Think, beyond pain, what a young woman can feel, forced to see confiscated a delicate body that the assaults of infernal evil transforms day after day into a land of desolation. The position and size of the abscesses often require the use of surgery to incise, so that their sanious content does not spread to poison the body with, in bonus, new scars reminiscent of the craters left by shells on a battlefield.

Everything is good to escape confinement and torture inflicted by this infernal illness that is the Verneuil's disease. Left to itself, the patient turns to solutions within reach as I did myself: *"The morphine-based analgesics"*. But in this troubled world, all has a price; these analgesics disrupt the body, but also the mind, widening areas of damage. - Left to itself, the disease spreads. I am lucky, in my misfortune, to be able to rely on my family and my companion who takes part in my ordeal. His presence with me is a blessing, and I say this here as a token of my gratitude because his generosity, my companion combines modesty that make him experience discomfort in any form of thanks. As he said once and for all: "I love you, and that is enough!"- The merit of my family environment, my companion, the presence of a few friends who remained attached to me, gives me the privilege to escape from time to time by releasing the overflow of what I endure. Although it is almost impossible to talk about his pain to others. - Pain ... These intolerable twinges which, starting from a point, irradiate to how deploys a storm lightning rolling thunder through the flesh. The flesh that it spins in burning them. Whatever the effort and narrative talent, it's indescribable thing. However, this right of appeal allows me not to sink into nothingness, and the destructive calmness of antidepressants. In 2008, because of the lack of results and the groping's of the medical profession, overwhelmed by a sense of abandonment, I cracked and decided to stop everything, not to swallow anything, not to be a Guinea pig for people who persist in inadequate diagnoses which, although ineffective, calm the prescribers, comforting them in the feeling of reassuring infallibility of their pontificating knowledge. Sixteen years ago I heard them, and that during all these years no one was able to put a name on this dirt that is constantly progressing in rotting my life and that of my family. Especially as the manifestation of evil remains similar, that I follow or not prescribed treatments. Meanwhile, the pain does not abdicate. It becomes more and more unbearable and I would come out on certain days or nights to scream under its onslaught. I'm not talking about my tears. The difficulty of expressing pain is only equaled by the difficulty of explaining the tears. Tears, these great thrusts that come from a heart full of suffering and despair, taking the eyes as an outlet, with the hope that by the distress of the glance they flood, they will be able to touch souls accessible to the pity. Alas, hope remains disappointed because it is in the silence of the night, far from the light, that we cry. Our tears are just for us, witness of our existence and our consciousness of being, despite what we suffer. They are the sign of our pain, but also our silent revolt against adversity. Although it is criticized on the level of ethics, it is more than once that the temptation has come to put an end to my ordeal by absorbing, as unfortunately many others, an overdose of analgesics.

I came to the stage where my life is only a daily battle with pain that increases its violence. I resist my best, but often the evil takes over, annihilating my morale, my energy and undermining the little good humor that still floats on my ocean of despair. 2009 - I start the year with an unprecedented rise. The outbreaks of large-scale abscesses last exceptionally long, and my doctor, Dr. Milesi, deems it necessary to resort to drastic measures. In my call to Dr. Chabert, surgeon at the CHPL Saint-Etienne for surgical treatment for what at that time was still called prolonged furunculosis ... It is the time of the preoperative consultation that the surgeon, who had to monitor me said: "My daughter, you are suffering from the *"Verneuil's deasese."* - My surprise at the statement of the name made him understand that I did not know what it was. I owe him the discovery of my illness finally identified by a correct diagnosis, after years of misinterpretations by all the *"specialists"* who had previously examined me. That is how I learned the existence of this infamous disease. Paradoxically, the fact of identifying my evil after all these years, had on me, in the instant, a curious effect; as a kind of deliverance. After seventeen years of wandering, I finally knew what illness I was suffering. It was almost in a state of euphoria that I returned home after my surgery, blessing the name of the surgeon who had illuminated my darkness.

Back at home, on all case dropped, in the paroxysm of excitement, I rush to my computer. The connection took only a moment, and still less to open my search engine and type on the keyboard: *"Verneuil's disease ..."*

When the screen gave me access to the site hoped for, imagine the shock, the confusion and disappointment that seized me on discovering that Verneuil's disease has no treatment. I was positively collapsed, broken, if not devastated, reading information indicating the evolutionary nature of this disease, which suggested to me that the pain I knew were only a first step and that further ordeals more cruel were waiting for me. My distress was immeasurable. I was trying to think of what could be the most intense pain that those positively infernal, I had already endured...

Small consolation, a statement indicating that the disease developed in three phases but, in any case, it's not mortal. Ah! Good, it's not fatal;

it doesn't kill. I would like to meet the authors of the article: Yes, Verneuil's disease doesn't kill. It doesn't kill the individual, but trashing his welfare, it rotten good humor, it destroys all forms of its future plans, it's opposed to a simple holiday forecast or that of a weekend. It destroys all the professional prospects; it puts a premature end to sexuality. It makes life a nightmare. I think that, from a certain angle, it kills in spite of everything; It kills what can be more precious than life, because what it kills is the joy and the desire to live. In this same year 2009, I learned that I have entered the "2" phase of the disease, and, as has been said, I have no other recourse but to live by accepting my destiny. I will have to continue to exist with in me this horror that will grow crescendo and with which I will have to fight for the rest of my life, for lack of the existence of a remedy. This fight resembles the game of the cat and the mouse, in which I will have to deploy at best the trick to slow the evolution of the evil. To do this, I must now compel myself to respect certain rules, seemingly simple, but which will modify a little more my freedom to act. Nothing complicated at first; I need only this *(I enumerate them in bulk ...)*:

> • Avoid using my toilet soap and the use of shower gel while limiting myself to natural soaps with suppression of cold water.

• Do not wear loose clothing so as not to cause friction that can irritate the skin. Select at least two sizes above the correct one.

• Dress with cotton, and use only this material as a bed sheet. Any other substance being capable of causing contact that generates eruptions. Let us try to imagine the effect of these restrictions and prohibitions on the mind of a young woman, whom the spirit of coquetry has not completely deserted. To see itself left to resemble a bag by depriving itself of all fashionable pleasure, that ingredient of feminine existence that belongs to the basic pleasures of life ... The only exception being in shoes that open certain latitudes.

• Prohibition of transporting heavy loads causing tensile stresses facilitating the appearance of abscesses. *(This is incompatible with the requirements of my work).*

• Do dress as cotton and only use this material as a bed sheet. Any other substance being capable of causing contacts resulting in generating breakouts eruptions.

Whether we try to imagine the effect of such restrictions and prohibitions on the mind of a young woman that the spirit of coquetry has not completely deserted. Be restricted by a bag dress depriving any kind of fashion pleasures, this ingredient of female existence that belongs to the basic enjoyments of life ... The only exception residing in shoes that open a field latitudes.

• Prohibition to carry heavy loads creating tensions which facilitate the generation of abscesses. *(Thing incompatible with the requirements of my job).*

• Avoid all forms of stress and emotional shock, *(while the life of Verneuil's victim is constantly subject to it).*

• Avoid fatigue *(As if it were something you could decide).*

• Do not swim in public swimming pools or rivers, gorges and beaches, except swimming and diving away from areas where sand can be hung. These prohibitions are not intended to prevent possible contamination of others, as this is not possible; disease is not contagious, but to eliminate any risk of damage caused by particle infiltration of Silica; These can be inserted into the micro-cracks of the skin which could then be infected. I could check the importance of the thing in the summer of 2007 when, finding myself in the Gorges de l'Hérault[12] with friends, I decided to override the regulations. I was going to regret it. The sun, the blue sky, the gentle warmth of the surroundings, the water reflecting the light of the sun like a mirror as an invitation to diving, led me to disobedience. The temptation was too strong and I thought that once would do no harm, and would have no consequences. I was wrong; Two days later, I was overwhelmed by an enormous thrust that doubled the size of my arm and that of my chest, all accompanied by terrible pain. As a bonus, two months off and the pleasures of last summer spoiled.

In 2011, I started to work hard to get a VAE[13]. It should be remembered that I was working on a temporary contract AMP since the age of eighteen years and that the absence of this di-

---

[12] *Hérault : River of the south of France.*
[13] *VAE : Validation of Acquisitions and Professional Experience.*

ploma prevented me from applying for a permanent contract. It was the period when I revolted against my illness, refusing to let myself be overwhelmed by it doing to me its disgusting things; A kind of playground allowing it to proliferate freely. With time, I finally perceive the image of my illness like a living being, a kind of demon taking possession of my body in full impunity, because of my lack of weapons to fight it. It was then that I started taking notes, which was a way for me to escape during a short moment to my problems, the time of a writing. I strengthened my need to escape the evils I endured by turning to beings even more disinherited than myself, whose suffering was above my own. The environment linked to the vocation of my company was not lacking on this point. This way of working had the merit of helping me to accept the horrible disease that devoured me. In October 2011, I finally got my MPA degree, which enabled me to be hired by the Red Cross in April of the following year. Shadow on the board, unhappiness meant that, during the same period, Verneuil's disease compelled me to undergo nine sick leave. I was desperate.

2012 was the year when as a result of my altered morals, my nervous breakdown reached the edge of the abyss, with days gone to cry bitterly, surrounded by people completely helpless to help me, my doctor decided to prescribe me Antidepressants. I did not know the direct and indirect effects of these drugs at that time. In the first week I had the impression that some bad fairy had made a void in my head; I had no brain; I was deprived of the tools of thought allowing me to know who I was. In spite of everything, I still retained the desire not to abandon my work, the people around me tried to convince me that my uneasiness would be dissipated by my occupations. It was a bad decision, because after a few hours I found myself in tears in the office of the director and the nurse of the organization to explain my situation and tell them that I ' Were note any longer able to work. By chance, I met the understanding of my head of department who, one day, found herself in the need to use the same drugs. Very generously, she advised me to go home ... - I followed the treatment for four weeks. Despite its side effects, it allowed me to endure the ordeal. I must say once again that my return to the norm was due to the support around me, to all the loving attentions that allowed me to recover quickly by suspending the use of antidepressants.

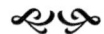

CHAPTER V

Living in spite of my evil

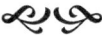

In 2013, the one that has now taken possession of me as a clean property *(If not unclean),* I speak, you will have understood of Verneuil's disease, strengthens his enterprise of colonization of my body. The major part of the conquest is made, it is now apt to appear in areas previously preserved, such as my ears. It is not an innocuous mutation because the humor associated with the saying *"sleeping on both ears"* reminds us that it is on this place that our head rests during our sleep. The presence of an abscess at this sensitive spot, on which rests our skull during our nocturnal repose, reveals a new form of pain, whose amplitude is opposed to the recovery of the fatigues of the day, so necessary to the patient. After nights of insomnia leading to little mornings where we rise stumbling with exhaustion, I fall on Anne, our Occupational Therapist, a formidable woman *(That exists)* who, listening to my misfortunes, Arranging for me to provide a mattress with a shape memory pillow, which proves to be a miracle by the relief it brings me. If I were to pray, Anne would be the object of my incantations; True Selene, Greek goddess of the night and solutions to problems. His generous intervention was for me a source of marvelous consolation.

2014- The year began with a dramatic event that created a terrible emotional shock. My friend Céline Kuzik, almost a sister by the extent and duration of our friendship, loses her mother in dramatic conditions. A woman for whom I was profoundly affectionate, and whom I met every day as part of our company, where she was employed as a service-woman, with boundless devotion, she was esteemed and loved by all. My sadness was founded in the sharing of the pain of my friend, whom fate had already struck three years before, and which now recurs, by making her an orphan. Living with her mother, the event left her alone and helpless in France; her only sister living in the West Indies, thousands of miles away. I lodged her for a few months at home, where the sight of his distress was torture to me, because I was unable to help her. I am unable to forget the moments of this distress. AMP like me, the equivalence of our occupations was a cement to our friendship. Unable to endure the new state of things, Celine decided to join the West Indies, leaving me a little more alone in my ordeal, which her attachment had often helped relieve. I was deeply shaken by this misfortune and all these added emotions ended up undermining my morale. I collapsed at the loss of my friend, although understanding her decision to go away by abandoning her place of life, become for her place of death. While I rejoiced for her choice of change for her salutary, the days that followed her departure were for me the time of tears. With Celine, I was losing another myself.

The mention of the drama of Celine is not unrelated to my disease, which is known to be prone to be stimulated by anything that is akin to stress. That did not fail, and I began to multiply the crises by developing abscesses to repetition, appearing little by little on my anatomy, ending with two months of work stoppage.

In the face of my discomfort, my attending physician, always Dr. Milési, did not disarm, and advised me to meet with the doctor of labor affiliated with my company, to inform me of the possibility to convert a fraction of my time of activity to disability, because of the impossibility for a wearer of Verneuil's disease to be employed full-time. According to his advice, I took the recommended appointment, during which the doctor who received me confirmed the validity of my request, informing me that due to my type of occupation and the nature of my illness, she immediately made the necessary arrangements for filing an application for invalidity. She explained that this request was for a half-time work agreement, with half the remaining price charged by the Health Insurance. Thanks to the diligence and dedication of this physician, I obtained this agreement in June. - Although it may seem surprising, what rejoiced me in the success of my approach was not to obtain a half-day of freedom, but the preservation of my job which was dear to my heart; Thanks to him, my life kept a meaning, my days would not happen to mop me by relenting my problems, lulled by sighs watered with my tears.

Being not at one additional bad new, I learned that the last events that I had just lived, causing a deep stress, had made me cross the last level of the disease called *"Phase 3"*. The news touched me deeply. I had fought so hard; I had struggled so hard over the past few years to postpone this change of area which would make me aware of new sufferings, which I was told would be more terrible than those I had already endured. It was hard for me to imagine what these new sufferings, these new pains, could be, more painful than those I had known. As a result of this announcement, my sadness and despair were renewed. God, it will never end? The *"No"* coming as the only answer to my question to heaven, my distress was greater. Especially as this pitiless adversary represented by the disease of Verneuil would benefit from my depression to attack me more brutally. I had little time to enjoy my access to my new half-time situation. As early as the 15th of July, a monstrous abscess began to be built. The month was not over, my arm and my right breast swelled, once more, in proportions hardly to be believed, doubling literally in volume, made more impressive by an inflammation of which one can say is that it was spectacular. At the beginning of the new offensive of my old enemy, I thought I was confronted with a painful abscess certainly, but, after all, routine, due to an appearance in the same places, and I thought that my twenty years of antecedents had prepared me. I must point out to the untrained persons that, by their repetition, the abscesses of those whom I shall call *"Verneuillés,"* end by affecting the skin, the thickness of which diminishes by facilitating the breakthrough of the anthrax. An evil for a good from a certain point of view... But, the reality was quite different; where I waited for a benign abscess, generating a supportable pain to which I was prepared, which, after the proper care, would disappear after a few days by piercing by itself, I felt the throbbing rise of a hideous mass. I had the feeling of being invaded by one of these sci-fi monsters, an *"Alien"* who slowly took possession of me. This abscess of another type developed deep in the heart of my flesh, engendering burns which, from day to day, increased in crescendo. Without admitting that I was apprehensive, I knew that this intruder of a new kind was going to lead me once more to the operating table because, by his volume, which I felt his presence in, I was aware that it could never be reabsorbed in the usual forms. I will not escape surgical excision. I did not want to be operated in August and, contrary to all expectations, I kept the utopian hope that the inflammation would eventually ease away from the spectrum of the operating room. I clung, supported by analgesics Morphine type. After 20 days of daily injections of *Rocephine (Antibiotic),* my right arm and my chest had depleted. This respite permitted me, exceptionally, to take holidays with my companion. Thus we set out for an escape of a few days in the south of France, in order to enjoy the sun and the sea, that exception which was allowed me under the prescribed conditions. I was all the happier because the sea baths made me crazy. The fact was verified by coming home with an arm and a chest completely restored, I was at the top of my relative happiness. However, hidden in the folds of my being, my invading *"Alien"* was watching. Stuck in the depths of myself, I felt it like a vampire sentinel waiting for his time. I knew he would not give up.

I resumed work in mid-September, holding firm, counting each day as a victory over the evil that was brewing, in order to arrive at the beginning of October, when I had to leave in the course of my work, for a training in Lyon, in view of obtaining a qualification endowing me with the knowledge authorizing the animation of a *"memory workshop"*; A realization that I wanted to set up with two residents with which I was involved in the project. As long as a maternal gestation, *(There were nine months I waited),* this formation was close to my heart. Alas, all the tensions I had experienced ended up presenting their bill. I was suddenly overwhelmed by a major crisis that required an emergency surgery.

I was rather confident at the prospect of a return to the operating table because I knew that I was in the hands of a practitioner in whom I had faith, as he was Dr. Chabert to whom, already, I owed so much. It was a real team for months, because the physician, doctor of labor department who had helped me so much in my efforts to obtain my invalidity, was none other than his wife. The date of the intervention was fixed on October 16, 2014. During my stay at the *"Surgery bloc"*, I was entitled to a beautiful, large and deep excision, the trace of which extended my collection of scars worthy of appearing in an anatomical cabinet.

Paradoxically, it was not the surgical part that I feared because, placed under anesthesia, the patient does not feel pain during the procedure. What I was afraid of was postoperative care. Contrary to previous interventions, the one I had to undergo left me a deeper and wider opening that would require the laying of wicks which I had already experienced the painful aspects. Relying on my previous experience, I had no idea what my new ordeal was going to be. I would have liked to have new words to express the suffering I felt during my first days of care. I have only to mention the terms *"Torture"* - *Tearing* - *Calvary* - Why such sufferings does have to exist ? It's inhuman.

Without prejudice to post-operative nursing personnel, I cannot help wondering how it is that, in a world as advanced as ours, it is still possible to suffer so much for post-operative care at home, is this a prevention or a simple follow-up of the pain? The nature of the words here does not matter. In spite of everything, I cannot exaggerate complaining, for I have the considerable privilege of being accompanied by a team of two nurses at home who, beyond their sympathetic approach, exercise their profession competently, provided that I have quality to judge, but in addition, with great care. The repetition of their visits ended up making me friends. Fabienne and David, these are the names of these guardian angels of a new kind, contribute to the relief of my sufferings by the passion that they bring to the exercise of their profession, and in particular by the compassion and empathy of which They surround those they care for with meritorious professionalism; the good mood as a bonus. It is a great opportunity for me to have them.

Without going into tedious descriptions, I would say that the first days of care consisted of the removal of the dressing. Then the extraction of the wick deeply engaged in the flesh *(The operative wound is kept open to drain the pus)*, before the placement of a clean wick which marks the time of hell of the operation preceding the application of plaster to protect what cannot otherwise be called wound.

The following days took a military tour: 9:30 am Wake up and up, when the night had gone well ... - 10:00 am: Like a cocaine addict, I shoot me with two *Acti-Skenan*, presumed conditioning to prevent pain, *(To take two hours before nurses arrive)*. These two hours of waiting between the medication and the arrival of the nurses plunge me into anxiety, so great is my apprehension of what I will have to endure. I have a stomach knotted and nausea at the thought of what is waiting for me. To say how much my apprehension is great, my caregivers will later remark that my portal has always been locked in the period of painful care and that, surprised, they then found it open, once the difficult period elapsed. As if, unconsciously, I had tried to delay the fateful moment.

We ring the gate. The nurses are there. The poor are almost crestfallen in knowing what they are going to do to me; they draw heads which, by themselves, suffice to reveal the difficulty of their mission. Exercising a profession whose vocation is to relieve their fellow men, the idea of making them suffer does not leave them indifferent; which is to their credit. After completing the treatments, I experience deeply painful swellings in the arm, whose will continue until late in the night, only diminishing in the morning. My respite, alas, will only be short-lived, for the same scenario will have to be repeated with the requirement of a daily change of the wicks. Pain, this old companion of my life, will eventually become bearable by the habituation that can give more than twenty years of endurance. Over time, my body, as well as my mind, became familiar with the pain. I verify this by the fact that at the very beginning a single abscess required the systematic use of an analgesic, whereas today I sometimes go to my work with two, when it is not three abscesses, without taking painkiller.

The forty-sixth day was that of my deliverance, with the laying of the last wick *(the last for this time)*. My relief was such, that if my means had permitted me, I would have sprinkled the champagne. The gaping wound, which the surgeon had left open to drain the pus, had eventually filled with a substitute flesh. All that remained was the surface scar. The treatment of the open wound had gradually replaced the wick with a greasy tulle, intended to prevent the obturating compress of the orifice to stick to the flesh. My healing was going well, and I could be happy with the complications that others were experiencing, namely, one or more abscesses that could reform before the wound was completely closed.

At this stage, several days, if not weeks, will still be necessary to achieve complete cicatrizing with closure of ulcerations. Time will again be necessary for a thickening of the tissues with a view to sufficiently attenuate the sensitivity of the scars, allowing movement and friction caused by clothing. - The image may seem libertine but, with the years, the panties have become unbearable. If I ventured to wear them, the elastics would inevitably provoke, in a few hours, new inflammatory flares. As far as brassieres are concerned, I do not know how long it will take to support them, although I choose the most suitable models, if they exist, such as those with wide shoulder straps And cotton. The end result is a premature use of the wardrobe of my grandmother, devoid of any fuzzy fantasy.

The ideal clothing with Verneuil's disease, would reside in the adoption of the costume of Adam and Eve residing on a desert island, if not in a naturist camp; although, in this case, good souls would probably ask us to dress for provocations consecutive to the ugliness of our scars.

During my work stoppages, I immerse myself in *"the web of the net"*, wandering on the hunt for comfort. How, you will say, since there is no remedy? I will reply that in this process my quest is that of all those who suffer from the same evil, with the hope of finding by their contact, or through their testimonies, the comfort by the sharing of the same experience, the sharing of the same ordeal. Regardless of this, there are on the 'Net' advice and remedies of good woman, some of which occasionally provide one off relief. I find there recipes to relieve all the additional ailments of everyday life: Reduction of the body scars, comfort of the soul, resorption of stress by Yoga, or relaxation by the coloring for adults, discovered on a site and Succeeds very well. The essential thing being to get out of the throes of my isolation by never remaining unoccupied; through exchanges about the sharing of the evil that I suffer, with other people who are also victims. Indeed, with whom can I best speak with a chance to be understood, if not with those who are going through the same ordeal?

Sometimes I joke, in spite of my heavy heart, knowing that I would have difficulty in making understand my suffering, for lack of being able to explain it to the people of my entourage who, at the human level, would eventually abdicate under the weight of a sharing, beyond their strength. As the English writer Graham Green said: *"Nobody knows how long can last a second of suffering. It can last the time of purgatory or all eternity."*

My days were spent in a rhythm that would have been appreciated by the schoolteacher of a nineteenth-century school: Waking up, often after a tormented night - Getting up - Shooting - Suffer - continuing the day on this rhythm. After my last operation, three weeks were necessary before I could reduce the morphine, and two more to suspend its use.

This year 2014 marked a turning point in my life. Heir to a playful nature, I feel that the accumulation of ordeals kills me slowly. Although I am inspired by the reed that bends under the breath of the hurricane, it is more and more difficult for me to straighten out when the storm goes away.

The phase "3" of the disease, in which I have just entered, sees it multiply its assaults, as if it foresaw the outcome of this battle of which it knows that it will emerge victorious. I feel invaded and, at times, overwhelmed by the anxiety of knowing how my life will end. In what state of physical and mental disrepair will I be in the final stage? Today I am already half a woman with a disability of level "1" to 50%. The time is near when the progress of evil will take away the half that remains to me by forcing me to 100% of the disability level " 2 ". - Tell me that, soon, I will no longer be useful to society by my inability to work ... My ideas swirl, giving me the impression of a drowning person who would desperately tend a hand toward a helping soul. Hand that nobody comes to grasp. I hear more and more talk of the use of antidepressants. This is another matter of concern, considering that 50% of people with Alzheimer's disease were subjected to it before sinking into their world of grisaille. All these thoughts agitate me, which I cannot share, because I cannot invite my entourage and my friends to the spectacle of my shadow's theater...

The look of others ... What will I not do to avoid it? The apprehension associated with it creates interdictions for me; thus, I cannot allow myself the wearing of a " tank top ", as I used to do sports or do some work. When today I sometimes wear one, I cover it modestly with a short-sleeved shirt. Gone are the days of the little summer dresses with bridles, so pleasant to wear for long walks in the holidays time. This garment, which, in true communion with nature, allowed me to enjoy the soft caress of the breeze coming from the sea. Today, I reserve it at home, far from prying eyes. A meager compensation is granted to me, by the exercise of a profession in which people, familiar with the suffering of others, have learned not to judge, by acquiring the ability to put themselves in the shoes of others. In my moments of distress, I have a system of S.O.S. My family and my close friends are aware of my miseries, I have the ability to mobilize them. A simple phone call or a small S.M.S, will always find two or three generous musketeers ready to enlist to answer my call. If not, I use a message on *"Facebook"* saying: *"Pff!!... I have my morale in the socks..."* So that in the minute that follows, I literally crumble under testimonials of support that are for me an immense relief. – *Cheers for Internet!*

My luck, in my misfortune, is to have had to this day the privilege, for it is one, to see my face spared by the disease. A privilege that allows me to conceal my evil by removing it from the morbid curiosity of the malevolent passers-by. I could not, without that, accept to expose myself to the pity or the expression of repugnance of all the *"generous good-thinkers"* who, you will forgive me, sometimes give us the feeling of enjoying our misfortune. It is as if some people come to blame us for daring to show in public our sickening ugliness. Let us invoke the cry of Christ: *"Father, forgive them, for they know not what they do."*

Combative in spite of everything, I force myself to be positive. Invited to friends, I sometimes find myself in crisis. To hide my condition, I turn to morphine, leaving my companion, Farid, to take care of driving the car back to the house.

Friends who know me and know how to detect the fluctuations of my condition, then install me in a comfortable chair by placing me on the adaptable surface of the ergonomic cushion that I always have at my fingertips. This cushion, guardian attentive to the preservation of the South Pole of my individual, of which I cannot separate, constitutes the ultimate protective rampart of my delicate foundation threatened by Verneuil...

At the risk of repeating myself, I would say that our best support is associated with the privilege of an attentive and devoted family environment. There is, however, one question: How far can this devotion go? For reasons that are easily understood, I do not want to become a bullet for my family and my entourage in which my boyfriend is included. When my sufferings are too deep, I sometimes appeal to his help to my aid to dress or put on my hair. I resolve myself to this end only in extreme situations where I can no longer stand, and when I reach the limit of my strength. The fact of having evil does not prevent me from doing what I have to do within the limit of my physical resources. Knowing that the thing would lead to nothing, I avoid complaining and moaning, convinced that it would only weary the people around me by demobilizing them. It is at least what I imagine in trying to put myself in their place, in the consideration of a human behavior. On the same level, not wanting to demotivate my friends by repeated refusals to their invitations, because of the constraint of my VD[14], I take on me shooting myself with morphine, and I end up satisfying their Invitations by asking an amiable chauffeur to convey me.

My ordeal in the management of my sufferings is increased by the pain of my relatives and especially my mother. I have no children, but my woman's instinct allows me, without difficulty, to imagine what she endures in a misery on two levels: her inability to relieve me and, more difficult, a direct or indirect responsibility in what I live, because of a genetic origin of the evil. Direct, if the thing came from her lineage; indirectly in the contrary case, by the feeling of a responsibility for having given me a genitor carrying guilty genes. We are, one in front of the other, in the manner of two tennis players who play without

---

[14] VD : Verneuil's Disease.

knowing each other, letting the balls pass without catching them, for fear of experiencing harm to their interception. I avoid putting my stress and suffering on her, while she, for her part, trying to hide her anxiety and despair from her inability to relieve me.

I often wonder if we are not wrong to prolong this play of the cat and the mouse which does not deceive anyone; Convinced that the retention of our feelings does us more harm than good, trying to bury our thoughts in the depths of ourselves where they end up gnawing us. It would be better to spread all this in full light, in the access to a frankness that would liberate our exchanges. Her anxiety troubles me, and the more time passes, the more she grows older, the more her concern grows. I work to de-dramatize the situation by not telling her what I really feel but, a mother has the ability to read on her children's face and I cannot deceive her with a smile of circumstance. Pain has its language which can be read on the visages as on the pages of a book. She has no need to see me to know where I am.

A telephone exchange is sufficient for the sound of my voice to supply the vision, and as soon as the doubt arises, I have, in the instant, the announcement of her visit. I find it very difficult to protect her by hiding my difficulties, as it is generally towards her that I turn when the ordeal catches me. – (*Nota Bene*[15])

I said I did not want children. This truth has not always been true. What woman normally constituted could assert with cold blood such a thing? I, and my companion, hoped to have some at the time when we thought that my disease was but a simple furunculosis due to the golden staphylococcus; Doctor having asserted to me that it was not transmissible to the children. That was in the *"2000"* when we even went so far as to try artificial insemination. Heaven, and I thank him, did not want to grant us despite five attempts. We stopped there. Today, I am to consider this failure as a chance and a happiness. If I had given life, my children would now be faced with the VD and its ordeal, like myself, with the difference that they would have known earlier than me what to expect, enduring an extension of their sufferings which would have ended my despair. I would have found myself in the situation of my own mother, who never ceased to tell me that she would give all she had to the world to be able to take upon herself the evil I suffered.

---

[15] **Nota Bene**: Undermined by anxiety about the future of the author of this book, Chantal, Doriane's mother died few days before Christmas 2016.

When the flow of morose and negative thoughts invades me; *"I have enough of living, I do not resemble anything"*, the presence of this real *"Alien"* who occupies my body deprives me of all the joy of living, I am exasperated by the suffering, and fatigue, then ...

I escape through creative occupations with the aid of which I bend my mind. Music is a great consolation to me as a stimulant. I move away from home; of this place which oozes the pain and the images of my misery. I am going to see those of my friends who maintain their sympathy and their support, become the land of escape and outlet of my martyrdom, and, at the same time, the witnesses of my torment. I have had enough of this struggle led into the shadow as if it was a shameful thing, when it should be meritorious. I protest against the fact that I am suffering undeservedly, and that I must also take care not to *"inconvenience"* the others. I openly want to tell people, *"In the name of a privilege of which you are not aware, you have been spared by evil. Do not turn your eyes away from those who suffer, for no one knows what tomorrow will hold"*. Instead of fleeing, join us in mobilizing you on our sides, so that those who hold power can carry out the research that will eradicate this evil straight come from hell. Passes for the adults, but do not let suffer children whose innocence cannot understand the reasons of what they endure.

"O God of love and mercy, if you discover these pages, please help this humanity that you have created, relieving its suffering..."

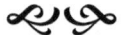

CHAPTER VI

Pilgrimage to the Damned

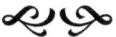

There is an excess of evil common to those who suffer; this evil is the feeling of isolation, that of a frightful solitude. The unfortunates who, during the Second World War, experienced the horrors of deportation, had the meager consolation of having around them people with whom they could not communicate by speaking, but who they knew to understand, by the exchange of a simple glance, the evils they endured. The disease of "Verneuil", like all evil disgusting, retains the entourage, leaving the one who is struck in the middle of a real desert. Suffering from this solitude, I decided to go and meet them. To this end, having not personally the faculty to communicate in foreign languages, I made use of the friend who helped me to write these lines which nature has privileged by the gift of tongues. With a pilgrim's stick, I went with him, to meet my sisters and brothers of misery around the world, in order to find the echo of my own sufferings with the hope that it would comfort me, if not relieve me. This is how I was able to speak with *"Verneuillés"* from several countries. I expose in my pages only some of my contacts in the United States and on the French sites. It should be noted that I presented the writings of the testimonies collected, identically, not recognizing me the right to modify them, even at the orthographic level.

I would start with Laura, in the United States, who discovered the disease through her son. I let her talk:

... It was through the connection to a website that I discovered the illness that my son was suffering from. I began by discovering that it was not the only one in his case and that the many people present on the site were confronted with the same problem. It was here that I was able to put a name on his illness that many of the doctors consulted referred to as *"recurring furunculosis"*. This disease, known as *Verneuil's disease*, bore the scientific name of *"Hydradenitis Suppurative"*. It must be said that at that moment, Paul had already undergone three surgeries and was in fourth instance. His condition was becoming serious. We did not know until then what to think, because he never had any juvenile acne. It all began with an impressive tumor on his neck, making a pendant, with the same horror in the area that served him to sit. Deeply shocked, he had stopped eating, to the point of losing ninety-five pounds. This at least had the advantage of relieving some of his pain by reducing the pressure on his buttocks when he sat down. The chance we had was to have, near our home, a world-renowned doctor.

Renewing our visits on the Internet, we put ourselves in search of anything that could bring relief to Paul, due to the lack of skills for the specificity of his illness. All the recipes were tried: daily time under hot water, zinc products, green clay, and so on. The last three results found were the only ones to give some results. Consulting specialized literature, Elaine Morgen's book, *"The Scars of Evolution,"* postulating that one of the causes of *Verneuil's disease* could be a consequence of our adaptation to the aquatic environment during the aquatic period of our evolution *(Why not...)*. Among the foods richest in Zinc, we noted the oysters. Paul was not at the end of his troubles. Anal fistula requiring additional surgery. Fortunately, his new doctor with thorough skills, could bring him some relief by the use in applications of his own centrifuged fibrin. My narrative could be prolonged, but it could become boring by the daily repetition of our ordeal...

Loretta: *(USA)*

... Loretta is one of the victims of Verneuil who, often, the soul in trouble, drag on the Net. She points out that Zinc and Copper deficiency can contribute to the intensification of crises. Sharing her own experience, she says fistulas are often related to constipation. *"I have,"* she said *"at the moment,"* a fistula in the coccyx, which broke out two years ago when I was only seventeen and still in high school. It so happens that my brother and my father experienced the same setbacks. My father suffered from it in his youth and was the object of a surgical operation which, fortunately, avoided the recurrence. This kind of inconvenience seems widespread because my brother was aware of several buddies who had suffered from the same problem. In other subjects, the coccyx appears as a zone of predilection for evil. Fistulae may appear, as well as very painful swellings which, as a result of a strike or a blow, may give rise to a wound requiring the pause of drains in order to obtain a cicatrizing . I experienced it personally by hitting my coccyx on a hard surface that triggered the swelling and a terrible pain. I supported this swelling for two years, before it finally opened without ever healing, requiring the permanent placement of a

drain. My only consolation is that this constraint has considerably reduced the pain. After two years in which my mother bothered me to see a doctor who looks after me *(she feared I had blood poisoning)*, I finally decided to plan a surgery to cut all that. When the surgeon prepared to cut into what was a two-centimeter opening in the center of a swelling that made four, he actually took away a huge piece of flesh and muscle from the lower and right of the upper part of my buttocks. The next two weeks were hell.

I now had to go to the doctor to make sure that my healing was right. After removing the stitches, he twice burned the flesh with liquid nitrogen to accelerate its healing. I had the good fortune, in my case, not to see the evil return and the healing went very well. I am now wondering whether the treatment followed at that time by the administration of zinc and copper at a high dose was not the cause of a recurrence of the fistula, which was declared a little later, Between nineteen and twenty years of age.

One of my cousin also had to endure an anal fistula about the same age, as did her brothers. They were both used to bolding their dishes with large doses of black pepper. I wonder if this is not the cause of their problems. The proof is that their fistulas were reabsorbed as soon as they ceased this practice. My own brother experienced an equivalent phenomenon. Although I am ignorant of the mechanism underlying this observation, I mention it in case it could help some reader to solve a similar problem.

Hélène (France)

Elena also had to endure the torments of an abscess which had engendered a tentacular fistula, as she tried to explain to us: I leave her the floor:

... I think it is necessary to recall what a fistula is and the mechanism of its genesis. The fistula takes shape when the pressure arising from the inflammation forces a passage between an internal organ and the evolving abscess. It can also cause a passage between an internal organ and the outside of the body. Similarly, a channel resulting from a simple anthrax can also be considered a form of fistula. However, the term fistula applies more commonly to the forced passage created by the thrust of an abscess directly digging a tunnel from one organ to another. It is thus that an abscess can spread its rot and infect many organs step by step. The infectious process will then be able to progress in many directions and spread over large spaces, colonizing fissures, cavities, and all voids that may be saturated. In women, specific morphology lends itself particularly to these polluting invasions. The fistulas are here liable to drill passages connecting the rectum to the vagina with permanent flow of fecal matter from one to the other organ. A fistula can also force a passage between the apocrine glands[16] of the rectum and the large intestine, with the possibility of an outlet opening through the skin. The disgusting side of the matter makes it understandable that people suffering from this evil refrain from talking to their surroundings. It is positively unbearable. It should be emphasized that the associations between abscesses and fistulas can occur on all internal and external points of the body. It is common for surgical procedures to cure them to be mutilating for those who use them.

Listening to and reading the statements of the victims of the VD are revealing of the community of expression of the people who are tortured by the illness of Verneuil, this evil disease. Gleaning here is the cries of anguish of those who suffer from my

---

[16] **Apocrine Glands** - *Secrete a lubricating material on all the points of the organism where lubrication is necessary.*

evil, I have found in them my own words, my own calls, my own entreaties so that an end is put to sufferings endured. Their clamor of revolt, if not of despair, will not have been in vain. The testimony of their torments will have helped me to bear mine. Poor consolation will you say that to know that others share the same evil, but a support however that of the discovery not to be alone; to know that there are beings who resemble me, capable of understanding what I endure without the help of words. Let them be thanked here.

To an anonymous from France: I restitute the writing as he wrote it. You the unknown, if you recognize yourself one day in this book, contact me because I appreciate your truths.

August 2009

The pitfalls of everyday life are the same for everyone. The difference with the others is a body which is treated as it is possible and which always carries new scars. A body that does not resemble what it was 2 years ago, all turned upside down after too many *"pushes"* followed by their operations. The electric scalpel, it cleans and it also digs, and it leaves traces ... less worse than a flare of Verneuil and much cleaner ... The scarring is long. And after? A remission? Maybe ...

or maybe not ... Uncertainty is the worst of torment; from hope to despair in the space of a night or a day of work. And between two crises, one notices that one expects the next; We forget to live really ... The friends are there, the relaxation sessions too, but in laughter there is like a crack, it's good to laugh but it does not erase everything ... Encloses within walls, physical as an apartment, psychological like a protection against the others. Only one does not live anymore, one waits always the next crisis, and when it is there it is almost a relief and a justification: You see it would have served nothing to open and to foresee and to engage, I would have been arrested in full swing and forced back to suffering and isolation ... I want to break this spiral but when?

To Hélène (Rhône - France): *If my testimony comes to the edition, I would like you to make yourself known because you are for me a sister who commune in the same suffering.*

August 2010 I just put out my hidden buoy at the bottom of the closet... *"It came back!"* It is well set, a little cramped, but debonair, reddish and paunchy, warm between the two hemispheres! It is curious as when everything goes well one soon forgets what it represents in pain and inconvenience unbearable! It's been seventy-two good hours that we cohabit and if at the beginning, I gave easily the change, tonight I cannot anymore!

For the past three days, I have been traveling to my work, falsely relaxed, with my hands in my pockets, and slowing down, telling me that it is better to appear more relaxed than ill.

The hardest thing is the endless meetings, where one must seem to be interested in stuffs of which one has nothing more to do so, the pain monopolizes the spirit. Especially do not move too much, have everything at hand; don't cough, even that, it hurts. And then get up three hours later - That's horror - not too fast, but not too slowly, with the air satisfied with a constructive end of meeting. Shake a few hands, throw a *"to Monday!"* full of enthusiasm, and force yourself once again, to tuck your stomach, clench your teeth and legs with a smile, and leave the room straight under the gaze of *"others."*

To cross the good girl who launches:
Hi, how are you? - Great form, and you?
And especially not to reach the answer because we do not care in those moments.

It's been seventy-two hours ... Tonight it's over, I just have to wait for my Alien to explode. Monday, I will not go to work, the meetings are over, they no longer need me and will do without.

To Clémence (Ardèche - France):

To you too, Clemence, I make the same invitation to Helen. Contact me if you ever read this document. Your letter is brief, but so revealing of what we endure. Your testimony is dear to me, a reflection of what I feel and endure. Thank you for sharing. Thank you for your language so direct and funny that it has come to make me smile through my tears..

... I introduce myself: Clémence, I am 26 years old and I am suffering from the disease of Verneuil. *"What do I do not know?*

When this conversation happens among friends, nothing abnormal in these cases, it is enough to explain with the right words what this evil is.

But when the same conversation happens between a patient and a doctor, this is a rather disconcerting situation...

So I start my story from the beginning:

After a very hard emotional shock, Verneuil wakes up with the firm intention of *"Arranging my behind"*. Of course, at the beginning, the name of Verneuil is unknown to all.

My buttocks, before being sick, were called boils; I had incarnated hairs, *(Ah! well, I'm hairy at the buttocks? Not Mademoiselle, precisely, they grow in ...)* I have heard that many times from people of my close entourage, the one still present today by family duty! People I will not quote any more out of respect for my children who, I hope with all my heart, will not declare the VD living close to those people who have the elegance of the Pustules they speak about! I fight for them too because I know they are not safe and that this world is brutal with sick peoples!

Finally, let's go back to my buttocks who have since traveled. They have miles as they say! And for good reason, they passed into the hands of incompetent butchers, So-called competent hand but who were ignorant. My Butt also got to know some unusual objects: A head lamp, a magnifying glass and it is left for a small turn direction: *"My Rectum Valley"*! What an adventure!

My butt have also known the scalpels which enter the raw flesh *(The famous butchers)* and then, the wicks that day after day are inserted in the holes *(those made with the scalpel!)* In order that the cicatrizing is done as slowly as possible...

And in all that, I spare you my howls, my cries, my tears. I spare you all the details lived, by me, by my relatives, I spare you what they live.

Still now and what is sometimes seen in their eyes, this tip of *"I don't believe you"*.

I spare you what sinks, sticks, suppurates, I spare you the smell of those bits of us who die...

The French singer *Guillaume Legrand* says in one of his songs: *"There is beautiful in hatred, there is beauty when it bleeds ..."*

Well, here I present my buttocks and myself, their owner, I present to you the Verneuil's disease, this disease that gnaws us piece by piece! I present my buttocks to this day, so that when *"One speaks on my Ass"* we know what it is!

And I lend my Buttocks so that every look that arises on them can said that beyond appearances there can be incredible sufferings, that this disease hides in nooks and crannies, and that it may seem invisible!

I want to stop those questioning looks, when we say, we are sick: "I am tired, I have no strength, I cannot stand this body" ... Look in front what we have to fight!! It's called *VERNEUIL!*

I want to try to make clear what your eyes do not see!
An angel helped me to love me, a dream like a journey where, with his fingertips, he showed me that for him the disease did not exist! A few words so that nothing is forgotten, a few words for him to remember, that an angel has wings...

For my husband, for what you are and all you already know: ♥!

I am only me to ask that things evolve but, together, with your help, we can make sure that the situation of the patients of Verneuil changes! For my Pals suffering from the Verneuil's disease, I don't want anyone to talk about Verneuil, I want to be looked straight in the holes of my buttocks...!

I want to be looked at, to see the bottom of the wounds of each and every one who carries

Verneuil with arms and who lives with these lesions and that our sufferings be recognized!...

My pilgrimage to the damned has brought me enormously. I returned as a visit to the Holy Land, strangely enlivened by the discovery of a universe in which I thought myself alone but which I discovered inhabited by these creatures apart that constitute the occupants of a land where grow sufferings and torments. Whether they are from France or from the ends of the earth, I have understood their language without difficulty because we use the same words, a sign that we belong to the same people of the damned. Like the animals of a herd separated by distance, we utter the same cries of pain, as would the members of a dispersed horde screaming at twilight.

Welcome to the club! Yes, we are members of a club of strict observance, where only the privileged bearer of the VD is admitted. We have our rites and our signs of recognition. There are no age categories. Admission is effected by evil. As *Clémence* has done with humor, we can exchange words that speak of the holes of our buttocks, without offending anyone. With the regency and serious attitude of the adepts of the naturist art, who can, imperturbable, be contemplated in their simple apparatus by appreciating, as connoisseurs I presume, the details of their respective anatomies. In our case it is not the sexes that distinguish themselves but the ravages caused by this plague of which we suffer and which makes us classify our veterans to the extent of their scars and the degree of horror and repugnance that they inspire. One could almost organize competitions, accompanied with honorary rewards, during which the most beautiful performances of the disease would be rewarded: Madam, or Miss whatsit, first prize of pierced buttocks; Mister Whatsit, decorated with the gold scar for a resorbed sex, eradicated by an abscess exceptional four inches ... As you see, I throw myself into lucubration's to treat my evil by derision; To show it that I do not abdicate and that I refuse to let it destroy me, retaining the ability to make humor, which remains, to this day, my only remedy.

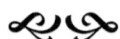

CHAPTER VII

Tomorrow Will Always Come

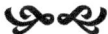

The thought of my future remains at the center of my concern, in filigree, the secret hope that a laboratory will find a cure for this dog that rotten my existence and that of my family. But things are changing. So, at the very beginning of the disease, I was terribly afraid of the approach of a new crisis. This idea obscured my thoughts and I found myself swept away in a great evil whirlwind that shook me to the highest point. Carried away to the bottom of my body, my illness was joined to a state of things which facilitated its task. I understood that very early, long before my illness was officially identified. It did not take many years to acquire the mastery that allowed me to dominate the situation when I felt the beginning of a new invasive wave.

My transition from CDD to CDI played a role in my behavioral evolution. Later, other factors came to join such as my recognition as a person affected by a disabling disease. At the moment I am speaking, I do not yet have the perception of the repercussions of the transition to a part-time activity, considering that the date of the event coincided with the date of my last major crisis which lead me to a new passage in surgery. I still have hope for a less emotional year 2015, which will enable me to recover a balance between my part-time work and the periods of crises allotted to my MV, who now enjoys a right quoted on my schedule. The stake is that this invading lady does not exceed this right. Among the encouraging signs, I enter my tenth week of convalescence, following my last resection. My arm is better, my wound has closed well and my new skin is thickened gently. One can say that at this moment, everything is bathed ... One could hope for anyway because since that night, Verneuil undertook an excursion in my lower floors, coming to visit without shame my coccyx and my pubis. This proves to be promising for the end-of-year celebrations that I will have to spend lying on the flank. Last year, at the same time, I joined my family at my mother's home and, as I was in crisis, I had to stay in my pajamas. This year, considering the amplitude of the offensive announced, the thing being in addition to the politic events, I think to opt for the *Arab djellaba*[17].

---

[17] Arab-Djellaba*: Arab coat.*

This beginning of the resumption of hostilities by my old enemy the VD creates me reminiscences, sort of balance of events with the inventory of damage, as it is practiced after the passage of a hurricane. My VD can rejoice with the results of its offensive. At the beginning of the disease, my abscesses did not pierce. By ignoring the pain, they manifested by a swelling that ended up being reabsorbed, leaving on my skin dark marks similar to a hematoma. Thus it began to affirm its conquest. I could, day after day, follow its progress by observing only those indelible markings which marbled my body, like the decorative moiré that the master gunsmiths of the "Manu" of Saint-Etienne execute on the metal of arms. I could, by this means, flatter myself with becoming a *"canon,"* but, I deplore it, it would not be that of beauty.

Over time, the abscesses increase in size and succeed in piercing without leaving traces of their passage, which are no longer manifested by a simple colored mark, but by an even more traumatic scar. Encouraged by the passivity born of my powerlessness in the absence of remedies, the abscesses now take it at their ease by holding meetings at the sensitive crossroads of my anatomy, realizing the feat of establishing scars on the scars. This domination produces painful results because, by settling on existing scar zones, the new abscesses raise the previous layers by forming outgrowths of the most hidden effect. Once pierced, past scars give rise to new scars resembling the tortured mounds of a lava field after an eruption. The image finds its full meaning, for it is indeed a question of eruption.

When the mass of the abscess becomes hypertrophied, surgical excision becomes necessary, leaving wide and deep tracings, creating a perfect war landscape by adding the trenches to the mounds and crevices. When the operation is perfect, no trenches, but a beautiful flat scar, which puts the original touch reminding us of the patches we used, in our childhood, to repair the perforated air chambers of our bikes. This is how I see myself gradually covered with spots that overlap and overlap because it is impossible to change the inner tube.

I am joking, but perhaps you will not laugh at my despair, which grows from year to year at the sight of the progressive and irreversible alteration of my body. My tears end up draining their source by the excess of their abundance. I have given up placing myself before a mirror; the vision of my physical decomposition becomes too unbearable. If I were asked what I felt, I would not hesitate to say that what I see in the mirror is not the image of a rottenness, but that of a mutilated being to whom my name would have been given.

Between the crises, I try to keep myself in the society that surrounds me, trying to live as normally as possible. My main constraint is to avoid the excess of fatigue that could revive an offensive of the disease. So when in my work, I am in the morning team, I sometimes impose to me a nap on my way home. It took me a long time to get there and especially to get people around me to understand my condition. First of all, they overwhelmed me with sarcasms like, *"So, you are taking a nap like the olds?"* Today, I know what I have ... During the holidays, when I feel a sense of fatigue, I rest systematically, without feeling guilty ... In any case, in phase 3 of the disease, It's my VD who now has the initiatives of my rest times. I respect his will, knowing that if the fancy of passing the limit would take me, I would cross the fatal threshold of a new thrust. It is enough for me that I carry something too heavy, such as carrying too many wooden logs to feed the fire-place, moving a flowerpot too bulky or too heavy, and others ... having paid the price of my apprenticeship of the limits of disobedience not to over-pass, I must be careful, although sometimes, all these restrictions exasperate me...

If I were to listen to myself, having reached the stage "3" of the disease, struck by an exacer-bated skin sensitivity, I would let myself go to live like Adam and Eve lived, understood *"furry"* it's the impossibility of entering the public space that prevents me from doing so.

In my moments of respite, I forced myself to go out, only for the pleasure, so legitimate for a woman, to go and lick the shop windows of fash-ion shops, even though what is seen is for the most part forbidden. Without making their pub-licity, the windows I am talking about are not those of the " *Gallery farfouillettes[18]"*, but those of stores like Gamm green, Casa, etc ... Although, given the situation, I did not have the Right to leave me tempted. I knew I could not wear them, I had to look for other distractions, such as visits to my friends, the latter choice being dictated by reflection leading me to think that I must Hasten to see them, because I may not be able to do so to-morrow; In case I do not have the opportunity to dress myself, under the pressure of a new cri-sis.

---

[18] *Rummaging gallery*

It is a well-established fact that women cannot live without expressing their femininity. As far as I am concerned, I may have suffered a little less from this principle, because my love of sport and a penchant for manly games always made me appear in a light a little tomboy; In the case of underwear, I have often used a boxer or a bra. As a result, the obligation to give up more feminine underwear did not cost me too much. This does not prevent me from imagining the desolation of the women who, as a result of the illness, have been led to mourn for all forms of *"fanfreluches*[19] *"*, limiting their wardrobes to an assortment that would not have disavowed their grand-mothers. In practice, the ideal is to completely give up the intimate clothes. That is to say the sacrifice.

Beyond the restrictions on dresses, renunciation concerns many other elements. For example, the formal prohibition of waxes and depilatory creams, resulting in the return to the hair clipper. *"Celebrating femininity!"*... Still glad that, with the help of technology, we find women's hair clippers on the market. The subject of clothing is also on the agenda and, as I have already said, the only allowed fantasy is reduced to cotton for extra wide models with fine seams...

---

[19] Trinkets

The cutaneous sensitivity developed by the individuals affected by the disease encourages the minimization of all forms of friction occasioned by clothing needs. My solution to this inconvenience: *Put my clothes upside down*, to reduce the thickness of the seams, removing all points of pressure likely to cause friction. Obviously, this does not lead to a summit of aesthetics, but it is much more comfortable and ease is felt.

The requirement to remove frictions is such that all the tricks are good to take. Of course, the result of this *"haute couture of cavalry"* does not jeopardize Jean-Paul Gaultier, Madeleine de Rauch or Paco Rabanne[20] but, based on the originality of the result, it could be made into an avant-garde fashion such as *"Design Rags"*, or, for the amateurs of Anglicism's: *" Rags-fashion"*.

The outstanding of all my vicissitudes give rise to a fear of another nature; that of depersonalization in which my *"self"* is threatened with disappearance. I would not want to become an embittered and negative person, an enemy of life that I would take in horror. I would like not to lose my abilities of native good humor, and the positivity for which I have always fought. In

---

[20] **Famous** French fashion designers

short, I worry about a change that would make from me someone else.

Throughout the world, there are people who are tortured to make them speak against their will under the influence of pain. I do not refuse to speak, this book is the proof of it, but I suffer, nevertheless, from tortures which render mad; Torments which would make me ready to do anything to make them cease. The pain often makes me bellicose and I become aggressive to the slightest annoyance, to the great confusion of my entourage. What is surprising is that I return this aggressiveness against me under certain circumstances. I will give but one example: When I am tired or, when I have been dragging my pain for several days, a simple awkwardness such as upsetting my cup of coffee puts me in a mad rage that ends in tears. My emotions in these situations reach unusual levels; It is thus that watching a sad film plunges me into floods of tears disproportionate with regard to the situation. I even melt into sobs when history makes an animal die. When I am in this state, I can no longer bear myself; I am on the look-out for the anomaly of a behavior that does not resemble me and which I also exacerbate.

When it happens that my morale sails close to the daisies *(What happens when the crises multiply in cascades and the pain does not leave me anymore)*, I am visited by morose ideas. I tell myself that the terrible evil that inhabits me will not only have no end, but as time passes, it will continue to expand by continuing its work of mutilation. I am surprised then to anticipate the future result of this work of undermining, trying to imagine what I will look like in fifteen years and the state in which I will end my existence. This projection in the future is not difficult in itself. I see myself more and more ill and deformed, subjected to physical and moral suffering, making from me a formless thing with nothing human, incapable of working and being loved. The gloomy prospect of what awaits me, traumatizes me to a point which makes me see the solution, through the thought, of putting an end to my nightmare by resorting to extreme solutions.

My strength, however, lies in my natural attachment to life. My family, my spouse, friends whom I can trust, constitute to me a force through which, up to this day, I have been able to resist successfully the destructive assaults of this scourge which has the name: Verneuil's sickness. Will it always be so?

Like all those who endure the martyrdom of Verneuil's evil, I live in the hope that a remedy will soon be found, but I am afraid of deluding myself in the present state of affairs because, apparently, no mobilization Is emerging in the circles of specialized research. A small glimmer, however, is revealed, considering that, twenty years ago, no one spoke of this disease and that for some time his name appears here and there on the Internet, in newspapers, on television , May be like the first fruit of hope. It is important that things should move and, for that, a mass mobilization of the population is needed, which alone can shake off inertia. The Verneuil disease has destroyed half of my existence like that of millions of my fellow men. I delight in the utopia that a remedy will be soon discovered, which will allow me to live the other half while continuing my work and not to end up as a pariah of the society, reduced to subsisting on the charge of my fellow men.

Life expectancy increases and the duration of the active period follows proportionally. Is it possible that the mass of the people affected by Verneuil's Disease is abandoned to a miserable lot when the means exist to help them by activating research? The progress of biology is now in a position to find solutions. Skills exist; Life expectancy increases and the duration of the active period follows proportionally. Is it possible that the mass of the people affected by Verneuil's Disease is abandoned to a miserable lot when the means exist to help them by activating research? The progress of biology is now in a position to find solutions and, as I said, skills exist; what we need is a will, the technical means, and the financing of a project. This expected commitment of the elected representatives is not the answer to a request for favor; it corresponds to a right attaching to their obligations; they have a duty to reply. They should come to see the children, the young, the women and the men, whose body is gnawed by an evil that covers them with deep wounds, which makes most of them skinned alive in the full sense of the term. Not replying to their hope, given their number and the horror of what they endure, would amount to a crime against humanity that would be a shame for our civilization.

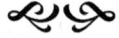

CHAPTER VIII

Verneuil's disease,

A Gehenna Prelude to Hell

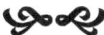

How to describe an evil that feeds on the multiplication of pain? Verneuil's disease ranks first in der-

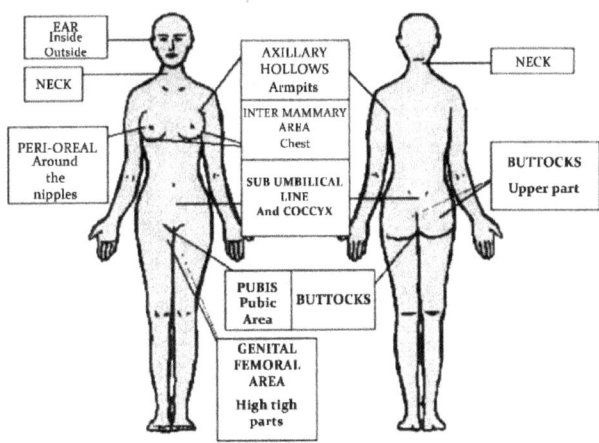

matological diseases. Three stages characterize it.

The first, the most widespread, affects 75% of patients, and the last, the most severe, 4%. I will come back a little later on the notion of figures. The aggression begins with red nodules, warm to the touch, sometimes suppurating, which manifest themselves in the zone of the armpits constituting a privileged place. The pelvic region, but also the torso, buttocks, genital area, face and scalp are also targeted. From the first stage, patients present varying forms of the disease that can generate lesions ranging from a moderate area to large areas of the body. What distinguishes the Verneuil's disease from a simple furunculosis is the presence of fibrous cords interconnecting the lesions. It is a chronic disease whose evolutionary process is caused by relapses, which can be exacerbated by fatigue,

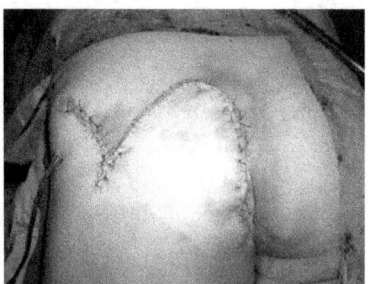

Scars four month after surgery

stress, any infection and, in women, the hormonal cycle. Outbreaks can become permanent in the most extreme cases.

Among other sequelae, the disease can have a psychological impact, due to the disgraceful lesions of which it marks the body and sometimes the face. Social life can be profoundly affected.

As if the dermatological alteration is not enough, it can be complicated by inflammatory eruptions in the joints which then become painful, swollen and warm to the touch. Imperative treatment of consecutive rheumatism is necessary, otherwise their aggravation may develop over time, until irreversible damage to the joints, regardless of chronic pain. The causes of the disease are not fully elucidated. Different hypotheses are made concerning local disturbances of the immune system causing inflammation which causes nodules appearing in more or less large numbers which in the most severe forms can generate large scarring surfaces.

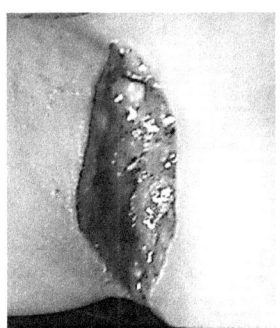

Wound left open for care after
removal of an abcess from the armpit

At the physiological level, it is not today of treatment allowing the cure of the affection by suppression of the causes. The only possibility is a decrease in symptoms as opposed to the infectious agents responsible for them.

Various treatments are proposed, consisting of local or general interventions using biotherapy.

When the nodules become too large to be treated by local procedures, the only solution is surgical excision, which is the ultimate therapeutic option.

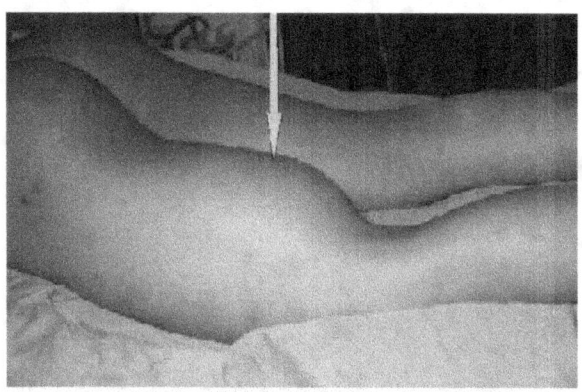

Enormous thigh abscess in the course of gestation

What should be remembered about Verneuil's disease ?

• It is an inflammatory skin disease with infectious complications.

• It is not contagious and, consequently, is safe for people who are related to the patient.

• Although it is a genetic disease, it does not exclude that a person without antecedents in his known ascendants could suffer it. Noting however that the risk of contracting the disease is much higher in the case of antecedents, given the existence of 35% of familial forms of the disease. It must be admitted that, in the present state of things, it may be that periods of remission can be observed as a result of various treatments: zinc capsules, trace elements, green clay ... But if one can; In a certain way, to *"control"* the evolution and the comfort of the patient with the poor means available to the medical world, such as antibiotic therapy adapted to the infectious agents present in the lesions. Recently appeared on the market, a drug: *"Humira"*, would seem to give results, subject to further testing. But *"Officially"* Verneuil remains to this day classed incurable.

Whether or not one is affected by this depressing illness, this veritable plague of Verneuil's disease, one cannot fail to wonder about the reasons behind the delay in the search for treatment. Whether or not, one is affected by this depressing illness, this veritable plague of

Verneuil's disease, the argument usually advanced to justify the absence of mobilization on orphan diseases does not hold here. Laboratories do not have to fear a lack of return on investment, because of the size of the market estimated at more than 4% of the world population; which, in gross figures, would give an average of 280 million patients. It should be noted that the reference statistics are very far from reality in that they were established in the West from the doctors who treated the disease; Now, it so happens that a great part of the medical profession, without ignoring the disease of Verneuil, seems to have paid little attention to it, with difficulties in making the diagnosis. What about the African, Hispano-American, Asian and Oriental continents. An in-depth study would certainly give surprising figures. These considerations show that the number of patients is ample enough to supply a market if the problem is approached strictly on the economic and commercial level. Why, in these conditions, states, so quick to finance wars, do not mobilize to stimulate research instead of giving priority to strategic weapons? Why do not our politicians, our deputies, elected representatives of the people, make their voices heard in the assemblies, in a concern that goes beyond mere commiseration for suffering populations, but to assert their right to life?

N.B.: The photos in this chapter are not images of the author, but documents extracted from medical documentation records. They illustrate, however, the suffering endured by all the victims of the evil. - I have not used my personal photos, many of which are more cruel than those presented, in a restraint of modesty which I admit childish, but which keeps me in the illusion of the preservation of an intimacy whose loss would deprive me of my status of human being, to make of me an object of pity or curiosity.

Not having the pretension to proceed to the drafting of a medical treaty on Verneuil's disease, or *"suppurative hidrosadenitis" for the medical world,* I did not feel the need to extend the photographic presentation of the horrors represented by this affection abominable. The few pictures which I have judged indispensable will suffice to give the readers a slight glimpse on the subject; My goal is simply to show the sufferings, and calvary, endured by those whom the evil has touched.

For those who want to help them, it is important to say that it is not pity or compassion that they need, but massive support from all to stimulate the world of research to do its work, finding a cure. Contemporary science has the capacity to do so and the solution lies in the mobilization of resources. Forgive me this parallel, but would we remain indifferent if we were told that millions of people are daily crucified and that the end of their ordeal is only a matter of money? That would be indignant; Yet this is what happens to the unfortunates who have been tortured by the Verneuil's disease.

At the end of my call, I feel the germ of evil reborn in me at this moment, signal of the new torments that await me. Two days ago, the VD, who had spared it so far, attacked my face. The envy comes to plagiarize the admirable verses of the French poetess _Rosemonde Gerard in her "testimony of love", saying, distorting them_ in the image of my scars:

... And each day that comes I suffer more, today more than yesterday, and much less than tomorrow...

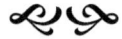

Table of contents

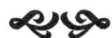

www.ingramcontent.com/pod-product-compliance
Lightning Source LLC
Chambersburg PA
CBHW071324220526
45468CB00001B/486